BEGINNER WALL PILATES FOR WEIGHT LOSS

YOUR STEP-BY-STEP GUIDE TO EFFORTLESS BUILD STRENGTH, BOOST METABOLISM, BURN FAT, AND ACHIEVE TOTAL BODY TRANSFORMATION.

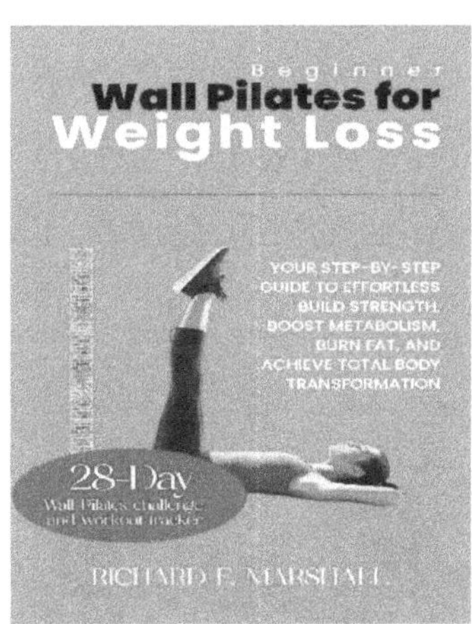

RICHARD E. MARSHALL.

GET ACCESS TO MY MORE FITNESS BOOKS

CONTENTS:

INTRODUCTION

Understanding Weight Loss

Exercise and Weight Loss

CHAPTER 1

Getting Started with Wall Pilates

Equipment Required

CHAPTER 2

Warm-up Exercises

Core Strengthening Exercises

Full Body Workouts

Cool-down Stretches

CHAPTER 3

Setting Realistic Goals

Creating a Personalized Workout Plan

Beginner Wall Pilates Workout Plan

CHAPTER 4

28-Day Wall Pilates Workout Plan

CHAPTER 5

Nutrition

Meal Plan Ideas

CHAPTTER 6

Managing Plateaus

CONCLUSION

BONUS: WALL PILATE WORKOUT TRACKER

INTRODUCTION

Pilates is a mind-body workout program established by Joseph Pilates in the early twentieth century. It is a low-impact kind of exercise that focuses on core muscular strength, flexibility, and posture improvement.

Wall Pilates is a type of Pilates that uses a wall for support. This makes it a more approachable and beginner-friendly alternative because it lowers the chance of injury and allows for a broader range of activities.

The use of a wall for support in Pilates exercises may be traced back to Joseph Pilates' initial work. He frequently employed the studio walls to assist clients with restricted mobility or injuries in doing exercises safely and successfully.

Wall Pilates has grown in popularity as a standalone workout approach in recent years due to its ease of use and variety. It is especially useful for people who are new to exercise, have injuries, or have restricted access to equipment.

Benefits of Wall Pilates for Weight Loss

Wall Pilates has several weight-loss advantages, including:

Increased calorie burns: Wall Pilates routines work numerous muscle groups at the same time, raising your heart rate and encouraging efficient calorie burning.

Wall Pilates helps enhance your metabolism by strengthening your core, arms, legs, and back muscles, resulting in higher calorie expenditure even at rest.

Proper posture improves your overall appearance, making you appear leaner and taller.

Increased flexibility provides for a larger range of motion, making your exercises more effective and lowering your chance of injury.

Low-impact exercise: Because Wall Pilates is mild on your joints, it is appropriate for people of all fitness levels, including those who have injuries or joint problems.

Incorporating Wall Pilates in Your Weight Loss Routine

Wall Pilates, when combined with a good diet and regular aerobic activity, may be a beneficial component of a total weight management regimen. Here are some pointers on how to include Wall Pilates into your weight loss routine:

Begin gradually: Begin with simple Wall Pilates exercises and progressively increase the intensity and duration of your workouts as your fitness level increases.

Consult a trained Pilates teacher: If you have any injuries or pre-existing health concerns, consult a certified Pilates instructor to guarantee appropriate form and technique.

Combine with other types of exercise: For a well-rounded fitness program, combine your Wall Pilates practice with other forms of exercise such as brisk walking, swimming, or cycling.

Prioritize nutrition: Weight loss requires a nutritious diet. Consume entire, unprocessed meals, as well as lots of fruits and vegetables and lean protein sources.

Set reasonable objectives, measure your progress, and locate a workout companion to help you keep motivated and accountable.

Understanding Weight Loss

Weight loss is a complicated process that requires knowing the balance of energy intake and expenditure. When we eat more calories than we expend, our bodies store the extra energy as fat, resulting in weight gain. When we expend more calories than we consume, our bodies use stored fat for energy, which leads to weight reduction.

Balance of Calories and Energy

It is critical to comprehend the notion of calories in order to understand weight reduction. Calories are a type of energy generated by our bodies from food and beverages. These calories are required to power our everyday activities, to keep our bodies running, and to create and repair tissues.

When we eat more calories than our bodies require, the excess is stored as fat. When food was scarce, our forefathers' storage mechanism provided a survival advantage. However, in today's world of numerous food options and sedentary lifestyles, this technique might result in excessive weight gain.

Expenditure of Energy: Calories

Energy expenditure, on the other hand, relates to how our bodies use calories. This includes the following:

BMR: The amount of energy our bodies utilize at rest to maintain basic activities such as breathing, circulation, and cell activity.

TEF (Thermic Effect of Food): The amount of energy wasted in digesting, absorbing, and processing the food we eat.

PAT (Physical Activity Thermogenesis): The energy expended during physical activity, which includes exercise and ordinary movement.

Achieving a Calorie Deficit

To lose weight, we must produce a calorie deficit, which means burning more calories than we ingest. This may be accomplished through two major methods:

Reducing Calorie Intake entails making deliberate decisions regarding the foods and beverages we eat. Choosing healthier meals, lowering portion sizes, and avoiding processed foods can all help to create a calorie deficit.

Increasing Calorie Expenditure: Regular physical exercise is critical for increasing calorie expenditure. Exercise not only burns calories during the workout, but it also boosts metabolism for several hours afterwards.

Exercise and Weight Loss

Regular physical exercise helps with weight loss in a variety of ways. Exercise not only burns calories directly during the workout, but it also helps with weight loss in a variety of indirect ways:

higher Energy Expenditure: Exercise raises your heart rate and metabolism, resulting in higher calorie burn during and after the workout.

Exercise aids in the development and maintenance of muscle mass, which is metabolically active tissue that burns more calories at rest than fat.

Improved Insulin Sensitivity: Exercise improves insulin sensitivity, allowing your body to better utilize glucose for energy and lowering fat accumulation.

Exercise can help decrease stress levels, which can indirectly aid weight reduction by lowering cortisol, a stress hormone that can contribute to increased hunger and fat accumulation.

Pilates is a unique method to weight management since it provides a low-impact, full-body workout that targets numerous muscle groups at the same time. This all-around strategy not only encourages weight loss but also improves general fitness and well-being.

CHAPTER 1

Getting Started with Wall Pilates

Before beginning your Wall Pilates adventure, it is critical to emotionally and physically prepare yourself for a safe and productive training experience. Here's a step-by-step plan for getting ready for Wall Pilates:

Analyze Your Fitness Level: Before beginning Wall Pilates, analyze your current fitness level. Pilates is flexible to all fitness levels, but knowing where you're beginning from can help you modify the exercises to your specific needs.

Consult your physician: If you have any pre-existing health concerns or injuries, see your doctor before beginning any new fitness program, including Wall Pilates. Your doctor may evaluate your general health and advise you on any precautions or changes that may be required.

Select a suitable workout location: Choose a clear, open space with a smooth, naked wall. Make sure there are no impediments or sharp edges that might endanger your safety.

Dress comfortably: Choose loose-fitting, breathable clothes that allows for flexibility of movement. Avoid wearing constrictive apparel that might impair your performance.

Gather necessary equipment: While Wall Pilates requires very little equipment, a few extras can improve your exercise experience.

Equipment Required

Non-slip yoga mat: A yoga mat offers cushioning and traction during movements, reducing slips and falls.

Towel: Keep a small hand towel on available to wipe away sweat and keep a comfortable grip throughout activities.

Water bottle: Keep a water bottle nearby to stay hydrated during your workout.

Stability Ball: By introducing an element of instability that targets core muscles, a stability ball can improve the efficiency of some Wall Pilates routines.

Resistance Bands: Using resistance bands to increase resistance to upper and lower body movements might help to enhance the workout.

Wall Space: Make sure your wall space is free and unobstructed. The wall should ideally be clear of decorations or jutting things that might obstruct your movements.

Considerations for Safety

When performing Wall Pilates, safety should always come first. Here are a few important safety considerations:

Maintain good form: Maintaining proper form is critical for avoiding injuries and maximizing the efficacy of the workouts. Seek coaching from a competent Pilates teacher to guarantee perfect form and technique.

Warm up your muscles before beginning your Wall Pilates program to avoid injuries and prepare your body for the activity. Warming up with light cardio, such as jumping jacks or running in place, and dynamic stretches is useful.

Avoid overexertion by not pushing yourself above your limitations. Begin with reasonable repetitions and raise the intensity progressively as your fitness level increases.

Exercises should be modified as needed if you have any ailments or restrictions. For individual adaptations, see a professional Pilates teacher.

Use proper support: Use the wall as support for the exercises, but don't rely on it too much. Maintain appropriate alignment and core muscular engagement during the motions.

Wear supportive footwear: Choose shoes that are comfortable, non-slip, and give appropriate support for your feet and ankles.

Take pauses as needed: Don't be afraid to take breaks when you're tired or need to rest. Avoid overexertion by listening to your body.

Set attainable objectives: Set attainable objectives that are appropriate for your fitness level and experience. Begin with easy-to-do exercises and progressively increase the intensity and duration of your workouts as you go.

Pay attention to your body: During the workout, pay attention to your body's cues. If you feel any pain or discomfort, discontinue the activity and consult with a trained Pilates teacher.

CHAPTER 2

Warm-up Activities:

Neck stretches: Gently rotate your head from left to right, forward and backward. This helps to relax the neck and upper shoulders.

Shoulder Rolls: Gently roll your shoulders in a circle, first forward, then backward. This aids in the loosening of the shoulder joints and the improvement of flexibility.

Arm Swings: Stretch your arms to the sides and swing them in a circular manner. Increase the size of the circles gradually. This warms up the muscles in your shoulders and arms.

Torso Twists: Stand shoulder-width apart and slowly twist your body from side to side. This prepares your core muscles for more severe activities by warming them up.

Hip Circles: Rotate your hips in a circle, first in one way, then the other. This helps to promote hip joint flexibility.

Leg Swings: Lean onto a wall for support and swing one leg forth and backward. Rep with the other leg. This exercise warms up the hip flexors and increases leg flexibility.

March in Place: As you march in place, raise your knees high. This raises your heart rate, boosts blood flow, and warms up your leg muscles.

Ankle Circles: Lift one foot off the ground and circle your ankle. Change to the opposite foot. This improves ankle mobility while also warming up the lower leg muscles.

Jumping Jacks: Do a few sets of jumping jacks to get your heart rate up and your entire body heated.

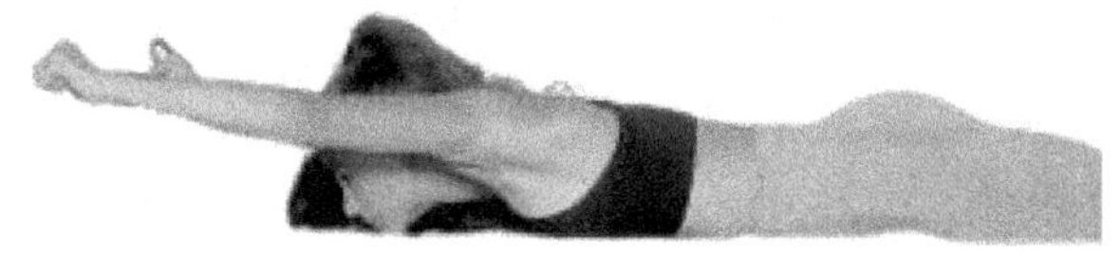

Core Strengthening Exercises

Here are some effective Wall Pilates exercises for strengthening your core:

Wall Sit

Target: Legs, core, glutes

Steps:

1. Position yourself with your back to the wall and your feet shoulder-width apart.
2. Slid down the wall until your knees are at 90 degrees.
3. Hold for 30-60 seconds with your core engaged.
4. Return to the starting position slowly.
5. Repeat 3-5 times more.

Reps: hold for 30-60 seconds, then repeat 3-5 times.

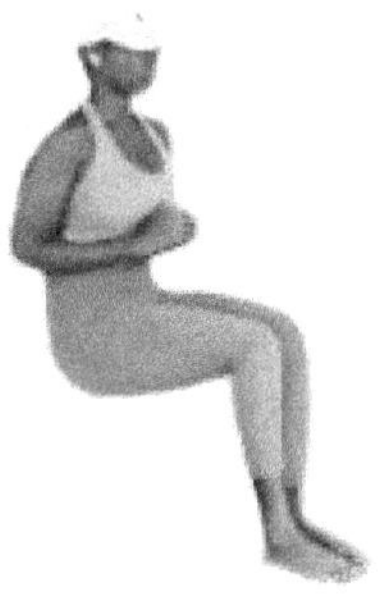

Wall Plank

Target: Core, shoulders, arms

Steps:

1. Stand with your feet shoulder-width apart and your hands flat against the wall at shoulder height, facing the wall.
2. With your feet, take a step back until your body is in a straight line from head to heels.
3. Hold for 30-60 seconds with your core engaged.

4. Return your feet to the starting position.
5. Repeat 3-5 times more.

Reps: hold for 30-60 seconds, then repeat 3-5 times.

Side Plank with Leg Lift

Target: Obliques, core, shoulders

Steps:

1. Lie on your side, forearm on the floor, elbow just beneath your shoulder.
2. Form a straight line from your head to your heels by stacking your legs and lifting your hips off the ground.
3. Lift your upper leg straight up towards the ceiling, using your core.
4. Return your leg to the starting position.

Reps: 10-12 reps on each side

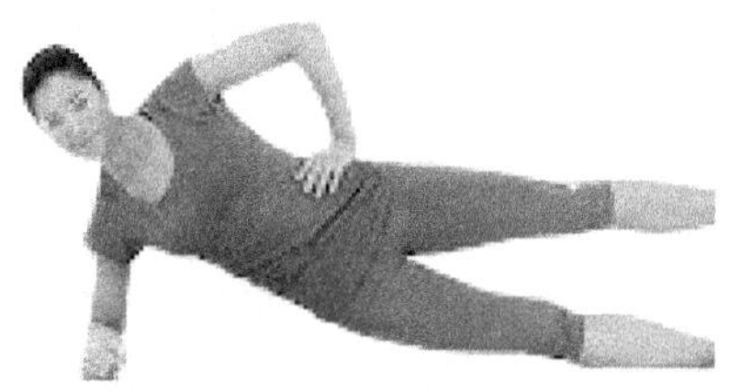

Wall Hip Rolls

Target: Core, lower back, glutes

Steps:

1. Position yourself with your back to the wall and your feet hip-width apart.
2. Tilt your pelvis back and press your lower back into the wall.
3. Roll your hips in a circular motion, 10 circles in each direction, slowly.
4. Repeat 2-3 times more.

Rep: 10 circles in each direction, 2-3 repeats

Wall Dead Bug

Target: Core, hips, lower back

Steps:

1. Lie on your back, legs bent, and feet flat on the wall.
2. Raise your arms straight up to the ceiling.
3. Lower your right arm slowly towards the floor while extending your left leg straight out.
4. Return to the beginning position and do the opposite side.
5. Alternate sides for 10-12 repetitions each side.

Reps: 10-12 reps on each side

Wall Ab Slide

Target: Rectus abdominis, obliques

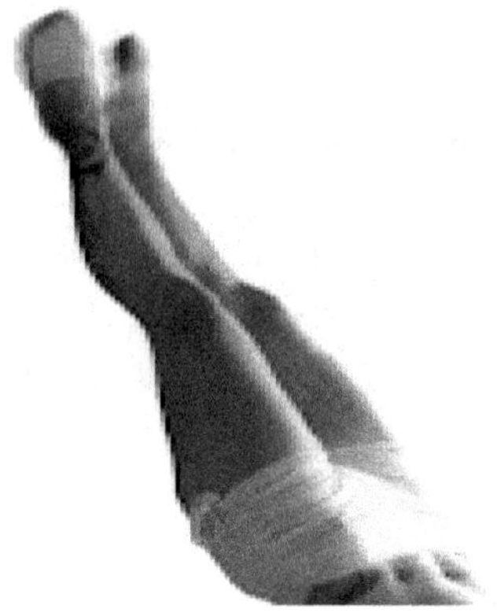

Steps:

1. Bend your knees and sit on the floor with your back to the wall.
2. Position your hands behind your head, elbows pointed out to the sides.
3. Lean back slightly, engage your core, and gently lower your torso until your shoulders are almost touching the ground.
4. Exhale and lift yourself back up to the starting posture using your core muscles.

Rep: Repeat 10-12 times more.

Wall Mountain Climbers

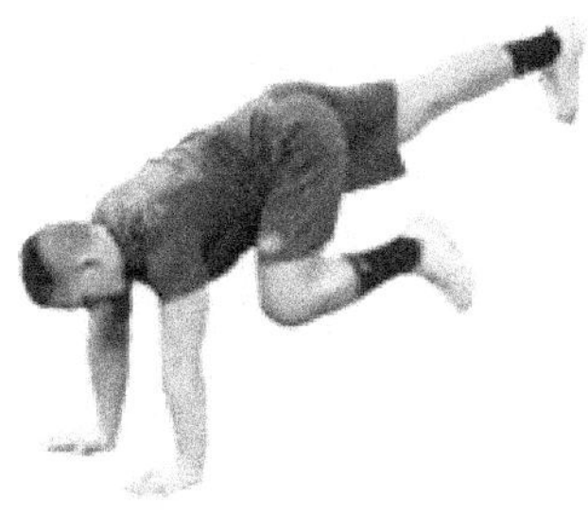

Target: Core, legs, glutes

Steps:

1. Face the wall and place your palms flat on the wall at shoulder height.
2. Step back with your feet until your body forms a straight line from head to heels.
3. Engage your core and alternate fast raising your knees to your chest, simulating a running action.
4. Repeat for 30-60 seconds.

Wall Pike with Leg Extension

Target: Core, glutes, hamstrings

1. **Steps:**
2. Place your feet hip-width apart and approximately two feet away from the wall as you face the wall.
3. Lean forward, your hands flat against the wall for support.

4. Lower your body into a pike posture while keeping your back straight and your core engaged, extending one leg straight back behind you.
5. Hold for a second before returning to the beginning position and repeating with the opposite leg.
6. Alternate legs for 10-12 repetitions each side.

Leg Abduction Wall Sit:

Target: Core, glutes, inner thighs

Steps:

1. Stand with your feet shoulder-width apart and your back to the wall.
2. Once you're 90 degrees bent at the knees, slide down the wall.
3. Engage your core muscles and slowly extend one leg out to the side, maintaining it straight.
4. Lower your leg and repeat on the opposite side.
5. Alternate legs for 10-12 repetitions each side.

Wall Squat with Ball Squeeze

Target: Core, glutes, quads

Steps:

1. Position yourself with your back to the wall and your feet shoulder-width apart, holding a tiny ball between your thighs.

2. Squat down into a squat stance, making sure your knees do not extend past your toes.
3. Hold the squat for a second, squeezing the ball hard with your thighs.
4. Repeat after carefully getting back to the starting position.
5. Repeat for a total of 12-15 times.

Wall Plank with Knee Tucks

Target: Core, shoulders, and hip flexors.

Steps:

1. Put your hands on the floor and your feet against the wall in a plank posture.
2. Bring your knees to your chest alternately, activating your core.
3. Rep 12-15 times on each leg.

Wall Scissor Kicks

Target: Lower abdominal muscles.

Steps:

1. Lay down on your back, legs straight out in front of you.
2. While maintaining the other leg up, lower one leg toward the floor.

3. In a scissor-like action, switch legs.
4. Perform 15-20 repetitions of each leg.

Wall Roll-Down with Oblique Twist

Target: Entire core, with a focus on obliques.

Steps:

1. Roll down, just like in the Wall Roll-Up, while sitting with your back to the wall.
2. Twist your body to one side at the bottom, working your obliques.
3. Roll up and twist to the opposite side.

Rep: 10-12 times on each side.

Wall Reverse Crunches

Target: Lower abdominals and hip flexors.

Steps:

1. Lean onto your back, bend your knees, and place your legs up against the wall.
2. Raise your hips to the ceiling and bring your knees to your chest.
3. Lower your hips without allowing your feet to hit the wall.
4. Perform 15-20 repetitions.

Wall Spiderman Plank

Target: Core, shoulders, and obliques.

Steps:

1. Begin in a plank stance with your feet against the wall.
2. Bring one knee up to one's elbow on the same side.
3. Return to the plank stance and alternate sides.
4. Complete 12-15 repetitions on each side.
5.

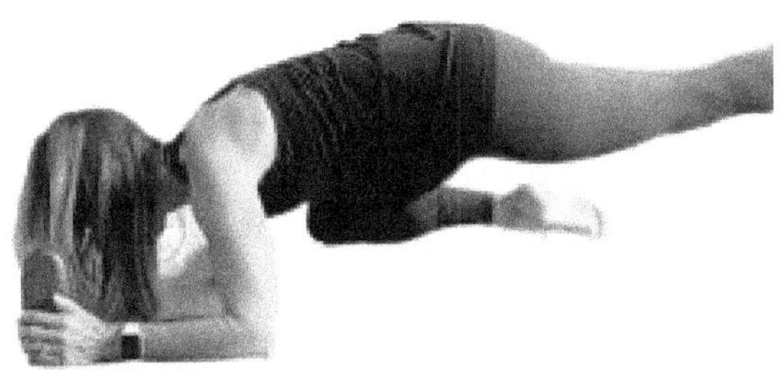

Full Body Workouts

For a full-body workout, try these extra Wall Pilates exercises:

Wall Downward Dog to Plank with Leg Raises

Target: Core, shoulders, arms, legs

Steps:

1. Stand with your feet hip-width apart, facing the wall.
2. Lean forward and position your hands shoulder-width apart against the wall.
3. Step back until your body forms a straight line from head to heels, imitating a downward-facing dog.
4. Engage your core and push your hips off the ground, going into a plank posture while keeping your body straight.
5. Raise one leg straight out behind you alternately, maintaining your core engaged and hips square.

Rep: Repeat 10-12 times for each leg.

Push-Ups on the Wall

Target: Chest, triceps, shoulders

Steps:

1. Place your feet hip-width apart and approximately two feet away from the wall as you face the wall.
2. Bend forward and lay your hands flat against the wall at shoulder height.
3. Step back with your feet until your body forms a straight line from head to heels, imitating a pike stance with your hands on the wall.
4. Bend your elbows and lower your chest to the wall until your elbows are 90 degrees.

5. Return to the initial position and repeat 10-12 times more.

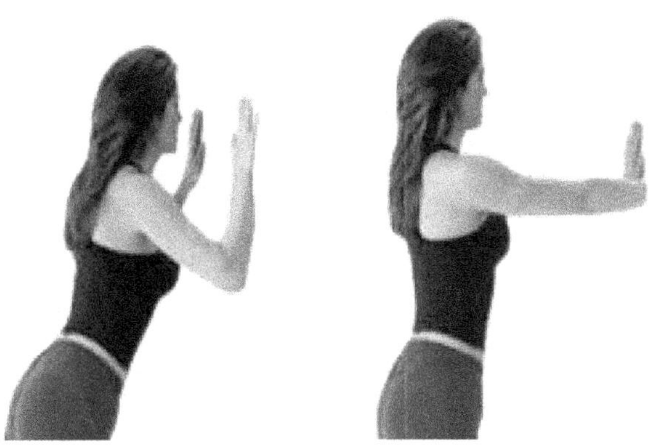

Wall Hamstring Curls with Calf Raises

Target: Hamstrings, calves

Steps:

1. With your feet hip-width apart and around two feet away from the wall, take a stance facing the wall.
2. Engage your core as you lean back against the wall.
3. Lift one heel off the ground from a standing posture, pushing your foot towards your buttocks until you feel a stretch in your hamstring.
4. Return your foot to the ground and repeat with the opposite leg.

5. After you've finished your hamstring curls, stand on the balls of your feet and do calf raises, raising your heels off the ground for a second and bringing them back down.
6. Alternate between hamstring curls and calf lifts for 10-12 repetitions each leg.

Wall-supported Side Plank with Hip Dips:

Target: Obliques, core, glutes

Steps:

1. With your right side facing the wall, take a sideways stance and rest your right hand flat against the wall for support.
2. Form a straight line from your head to your heels by stacking your feet and lifting your hips off the ground.
3. Engage your core and steadily descend your hips to the ground while maintaining your body straight.
4. Dip your hips as far as they will go and then push back up to the starting position.
5. Roll onto your other side and repeat on the opposite side 10-12 times.

Wall Plank with Leg Circles

Target: Core, shoulders, and hip flexors.

Steps:

1. Get into a plank posture with your feet against the wall.
2. In a controlled motion, circle one leg.
3. Change legs and directions.
4. On each leg, make 10 circles in each direction.

Arm Circles on the Wall

Target: Legs, core, shoulders

Steps:

1. Position yourself with your back to the wall and your feet shoulder-width apart.
2. Slide along the wall until your knees are 90 degrees bent.
3. Hold with your core engaged.
4. Make little forward and backward circles with your arms for 10 repetitions in each direction.
5. Repeat 3-5 times more.

Wall Plank with Lateral Leg Lifts

Target: Core, shoulders, arms, legs

Steps:

1. Place your hands flat against the wall at shoulder height and face the wall with your feet shoulder-width apart.
2. With your feet, take a step back until your body is in a straight line from head to heels.
3. Hold for 30 seconds while keeping your core engaged.
4. Stretch one leg out to the side while maintaining your core engaged and your hips square.
5. Lower your leg back down and repeat with the opposite leg, alternating for 10-12 repetitions each leg.

Wall Push-Ups with Tricep Dips

Target: Chest, triceps, shoulders

Steps:

1. With your arms extended and your feet shoulder-width apart, take a stance facing the wall.
2. Place your hands flat on the wall, shoulder-width apart, at shoulder height.
3. Rest against the wall and bend your elbows, lowering your chest until your elbows are bent at a 90-degree angle.
4. Return to the starting position by pushing up.
5. Lower your elbows even deeper, past 90 degrees, to dip your triceps.

6. Return to your starting posture and repeat 10-12 times more.

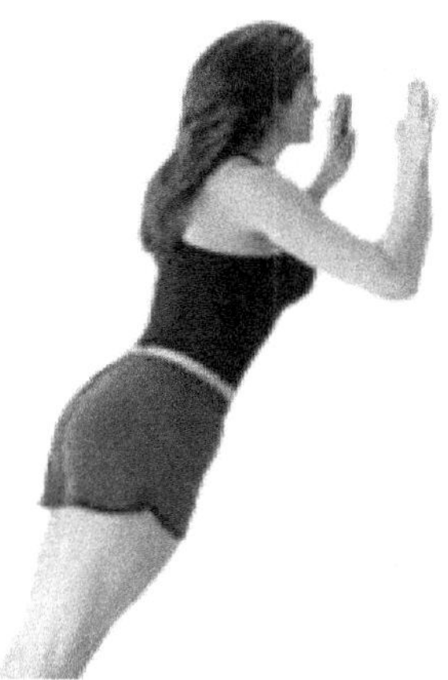

Wall Squats with Bicep Curls and Shoulder Press

Target: Legs, glutes, biceps, shoulders

Steps:

1. With your feet shoulder-width apart, lean your back against the wall.
2. Hold two dumbbells at your sides in your hands.
3. Squat down while maintaining your knees behind your toes and your back straight.
4. Curl the dumbbells up towards your shoulders as you squat.
5. Return to your feet and press the dumbbells above until your arms are completely extended.
6. Return the dumbbells to your sides and repeat 12-15 times.

Wall-supported Lunges with Overhead Reach

Target: Legs, glutes, shoulders

Steps:

1. Stand with one hand flat on the wall for support.
2. With one leg, take a step forward and drop yourself into a lunge, bending your front knee to a 90-degree angle.
3. Reach your other arm above and completely stretch it as you lunge.
4. Stand up again, dropping your arm to your side.
5. Repeat 10-12 times for each leg.

Cool-down Stretches

Here are some great cool-down stretches to do after your weight reduction Wall Pilates workout:

Standing Hamstring Stretch

Target: Hamstrings

Steps:

1. Place your feet hip-width apart and stand tall.
2. Hinge at your hips and fold forward slowly, aiming for your toes.

3. Maintain a straight back and slightly bowed knees.
4. Maintain for 30-60 seconds.

Seated Calf Stretch

Target: Calves

Steps:

1. Sit on the floor and extend your legs straight out in front of you.
2. Wrap a towel over the ball of your right foot and gradually draw it towards your body until you feel a calf stretch.
3. Hold for 30-60 seconds before repeating with the opposite leg.

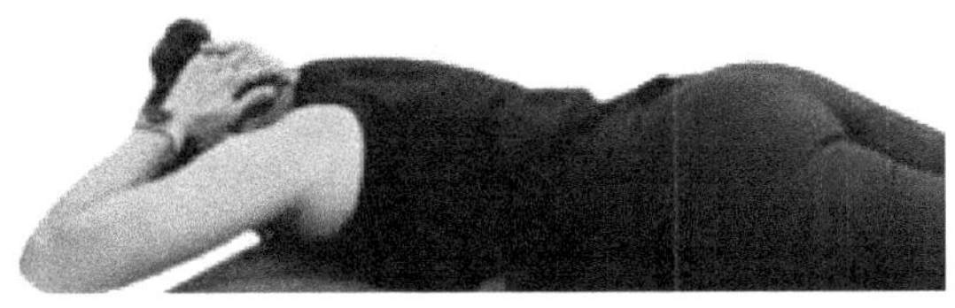

Quad Stretch

Target: Quads

Steps:

1. Standing on one leg, bend the other knee and pull your heel towards your buttocks.
2. Hold your ankle with one hand and bring your heel closer to your torso until your quadriceps stretch.
3. Hold for 30-60 seconds before repeating with the opposite leg.

Chest Opener

Target: Chest

Steps:

1. Stand tall, your feet hip-width apart, and your arms at your sides.
2. Hold your hands behind your back, palms facing outwards.
3. Push your chest forward and open your shoulders gently.
4. Maintain for 30-60 seconds.

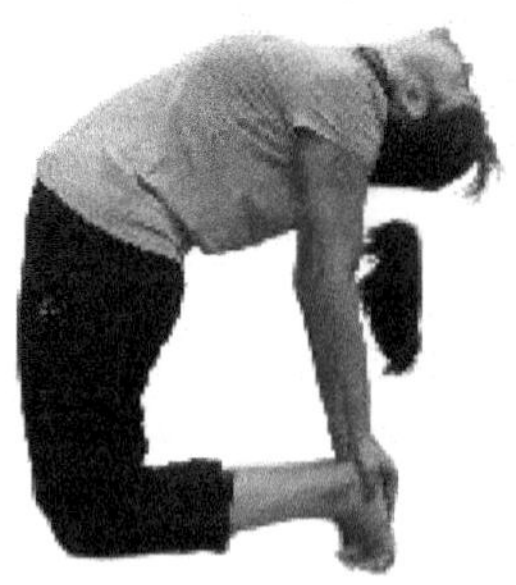

The Spine Twist

Target: Spine

Steps:

1. Sit on the floor and extend your legs straight out in front of you.
2. Bend your right knee and place your foot on the floor just outside your left thigh.
3. Twist your body to the right, supporting yourself with your left hand on the floor.
4. Examine your right shoulder.
5. Hold for 30-60 seconds before repeating on the opposite side.

Butterfly Stretch on the Wall

Target: Inner thighs, groin

Steps:

1. Stand with your feet hip-width apart and about two feet away from the wall, facing it.
2. Lie back and rest your hands on the wall for stability.
3. Slide your feet down the wall slowly until your knees are at a 90-degree angle and your soles are touching.
4. Maintain for 30-60 seconds.

The Cat-Cow Pose

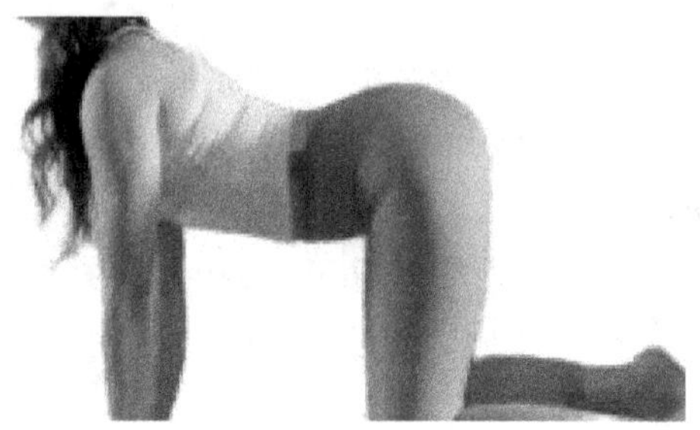

Target: Spine, neck, shoulders

Steps:

1. Begin on your hands and knees, shoulder-width apart, and knees hip-width apart.
2. Inhale and arch your back, lowering your belly to the ground and gazing up (cow position).
3. Exhale and circle your back (cat position), tucking your chin into your chest and thrusting your hips towards the ceiling.
4. Repeat 10-12 times more.

Neck Rolls

Target: Neck

Steps:

1. Sit or stand tall, shoulders relaxed.
2. Slowly roll your head in a circular motion for 10 repetitions, first clockwise, then counter-clockwise.
3. Hold for 15 seconds while gently tilting your head to one side, bringing your ear near your shoulder.
4. Rep on the opposite side.

Wrist Circles

Target: Wrists

Steps:

1. Stretch your arms out in front of you, palms facing down.
2. Slowly move your wrists in circles, first clockwise for 10 repetitions, then counter-clockwise for 10 repetitions.
3. Repeat the circular motions with your palms facing up.

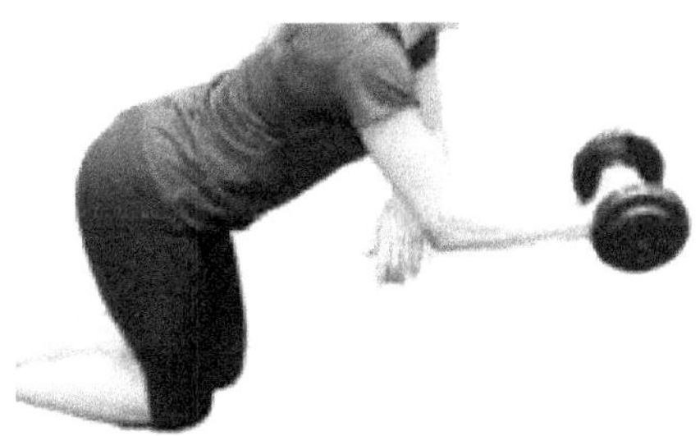

Ankle Rolls

Target: Ankles

Steps:

1. Place your feet flat on the floor and sit or stand tall.
2. Slowly roll your ankles in a circular manner for 10 repetitions, first clockwise, then anticlockwise.

CHAPTER 3

Setting Realistic Goals

Wall Pilates is an effective weight-loss strategy because it provides a low-impact, full-body workout that activates various muscle groups, burns calories, and tones your body. But where do you begin? Let's get into the details of creating a tailored Wall Pilates training plan that can help you reach your weight reduction objectives.

Setting Realistic Goals, It is critical to set realistic goals before beginning your Wall Pilates adventure. Long-term success requires a focus on sustainable improvement.

Consider the following factors:

Current level of fitness: Begin by honestly assessing your present level of fitness. Do you consider yourself a beginning, intermediate, or experienced exerciser?

Weight loss objectives: Set attainable and realistic weight loss objectives. Aim for a weekly weight loss of 1-2 pounds that is gradual and sustained.

Time available: Determine how much time you can devote to your fitness regimen each week.

Creating a Personalized Workout Plan

Once your goals have been set, it is time to create a customized training plan. Here's how it's done:

Frequency: For best results, try to do three Wall Pilates sessions a week at minimum.

Duration: As your fitness level increases, progressively extend the length of your workouts from 20 to 30 minutes at first.

Intensity: Select exercises that will push you while remaining doable. Priority should be given to appropriate form and technique above speed.

Include a wide range of workouts to target different muscle groups and avoid plateaus.

Warm-up and cool-down: Set aside 5-10 minutes before every workout to warm up your muscles and cool down with stretches.

Beginner Wall Pilates Workout Plan

5 minute warm-up:

- 10 repetitions of neck rolls in each direction
- 10 repetitions of shoulder rolls in either direction
- 10 reps forward and backward arm circles
- 10 wrist rolls in each direction
- 10 ankle rolls in each direction

Exercise (20-25 minutes):

- 3 sets of 30 seconds on the wall
- 3 sets of 10 repetitions of wall push-ups
- 3 sets of 15 reps of wall squats
- 3 sets of 10 reps per leg on the wall
- 3 sets of 30 seconds wall plank
- 3 sets of 30 seconds on either side of the wall

Relaxation (5 minutes):

- 30 seconds standing hamstring stretch
- 30 seconds hold per leg for seated calf stretch
- Hold the quad stretch for 30 seconds per leg.
- 30 second hold on the chest opener
- Twist your spine for 30 seconds on each side.

Monitoring Progress

Long-term success requires staying motivated and on track. Keep track of your progress by:

Monitoring weight loss: Weigh yourself on a regular basis, but avoid obsessing over the amount.

Keeping an exercise log: Keep a workout log that includes exercises, sets, repetitions, and duration.

Photographs of progress: To notice physical improvements, take progress shots every couple week.

Milestone recognition and celebration: Recognize and celebrate your accomplishments, no matter how modest.

NOTE

Consistency is essential: You will see benefits if you stick to your fitness plan.

Listen to your body: Don't overdo it, especially when you're just beginning out. Rest as required.

Make it enjoyable: Choose exercises that you love and listen to music while working out.

Seek assistance: Sign up for a class, locate a workout companion, or see a fitness professional for specialized advice.

CHAPTER 4

This 28-day Wall Pilates exercise regimen is intended to help you burn calories, tone your muscles, and lose weight. It includes a range of exercises that target various muscle groups and gradually rises in intensity throughout the session. Remember that consistency and appropriate form are essential for getting results.

Before You Begin:

- Before starting any new workout plan, consult with your doctor.
- Warm up by performing 5-10 minutes of mild aerobic and dynamic stretches.
- Cool down with static stretches for 5-10 minutes.
- Listen to your body and take breaks as required.
- Adapt activities to your fitness level as required.
- To stay motivated, keep track of your progress.

Week 1:

Day 1:

- 3 sets of 30 seconds on the wall
- Push-ups against the wall (3 sets of 10 reps)

- Squats against the wall (3 sets of 15 reps)
- 3 sets of 12 repetitions of wall hip raises
- Plank (3 sets of 30 seconds)

Day 2:

- Wall Lunges (3 sets of 10 repetitions each)
- Plank on the wall (3 sets of 30 seconds per side)
- Bicep Curls on the Wall (3 sets of 15 reps)
- Tricep Dips on the Wall (3 sets of 12 reps)
- Shoulder Press on the Wall (3 sets of 12 repetitions)

Day 3:

- 3 sets of 30 seconds hold on the wall
- Push-ups against the wall (3 sets of 10 reps)
- V-Sit Hold on the Wall (3 sets of 30 seconds)
- Wall Hamstring Curls (3 sets of 15 repetitions)
- Calf Raises on the Wall (3 sets of 20 repetitions)

Week 2:

Day 4:

- 3 sets of 45 seconds on the wall
- Push-ups against the wall (3 sets of 12 reps)
- Jumps with Wall Squats (3 sets of 12 repetitions)

- Hip Bridges on the Wall with Leg Abduction (3 sets of 15 repetitions per leg)
- Shoulder Taps with a Wall Plank (3 sets of 30 seconds)

Day 5:

- Leg Extensions with Wall Lunges (3 sets of 12 repetitions per leg)
- Wall Side Planks with Hip Dips (3 sets of 30 seconds each)
- 3 sets of 12 repetitions of wall bicep curls with hammer curls
- Tricep Dips on the Wall with Overhead Tricep Extensions (3 sets of 12 reps)
- Lateral Wall Raises (3 sets of 12 repetitions)

Day 6:

- 3 sets of 5 repetitions of Wall Downward Dog to Plank
- Push-ups against the wall with leg extensions (3 sets of 10 reps)
- V-Sit on the wall with alternate leg raises (3 sets of 30 seconds)
- Calf Raises with Wall Hamstring Curls (3 sets x 12 repetitions each leg)
- Wall Climbers (3 sets of 30 seconds)

Week 3:

Day 7:

- Arm Circles on the Wall (3 sets of 1 minute)
- Push-Ups on the Wall (3 sets of 10 reps)
- Pulse Wall Squats (3 sets of 15 reps)
- Wall Hip Raises with Single Leg Extension (3 sets of 12 repetitions)
- Wall Planks with Side Plank Holds (3 sets of 30 seconds each)

Day 8:

- Squats against the wall (3 sets of 10 repetitions per leg)
- Wall Side Planks with Leg Lifts (3 sets of 30 seconds each)
- Concentration Curls with Wall Bicep Curls (3 sets x 12 repetitions)
- Tricep Dips on the Wall with Skull Crushers (3 sets of 12 reps)
- Front Wall Raises (3 sets of 12 repetitions)

Day 9:

- 3 sets of 5 repetitions from wall plank to downward dog

- Push-ups on the wall (3 sets x as many repetitions as feasible)
- L-Sit Hold on the Wall (3 sets of 30 seconds)
- Hamstring Curls on the Wall with a Pilates Ball (3 sets of 12 repetitions per leg)
- Burpees on the wall (3 sets of 10 repetitions)

Week 4:

Day 10:

- Active Rest: Light aerobics or yoga

Day 11

- 3 sets of 1-minute wall sit with overhead reach
- 3 sets of 10 reps push-ups against the wall
- Single Leg Press with Wall Squats (3 sets of 15 repetitions per leg)
- Pulsed Wall Glute Bridges (3 sets of 12 repetitions per leg)
- 3 sets of 30 seconds on either side of a wall plank with hip twists

Day 12:

- Sumo Squats against the wall (3 sets of 10 repetitions per leg)

- Wall Side Plank with Leg Abduction (3 sets of 30 seconds)
- Wall Hammer Curls alternating with Zottman Curls (3 sets of 12 repetitions)
- Tricep Dips on the Wall with an Overhead Press (3 sets of 12 reps)
- Reverse Flyes on the Wall (3 sets of 12 repetitions)

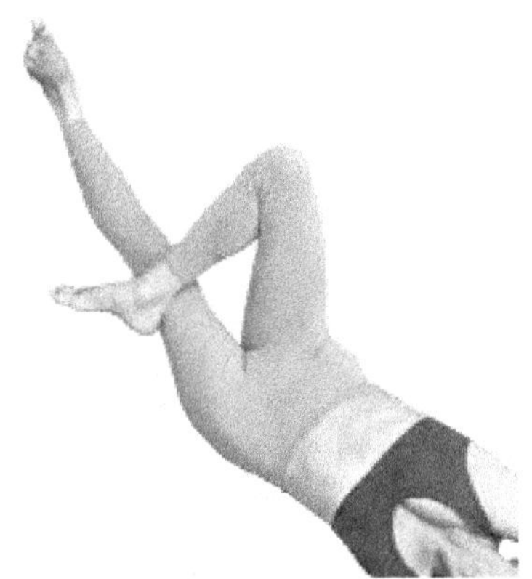

Day 13:

- 3 sets of 5 repetitions of Wall Downward Dog to Plank with Shoulder Taps
- 3 sets of 10 reps pike Push-Ups on the Wall
- Wall V-Sit with Leg Raises and Extensions (3 sets of 30 seconds)
- 3 sets x 12 reps each leg Calf Raises and Wall Hamstring Curls with a Pilates Ball

- 3 sets of 30 seconds climbers on the Wall with High Knees

Week 5:

Day 14:

- Light aerobics or yoga for active rest

Day 15:

- 3 sets of 1-minute Bicep curls and shoulder press against the wall
- 3 sets of 10 reps Push-ups against the wall
- 3 sets of 12 repetitions of wall squats with jumps and overhead press
- 3 sets of 12 repetitions per leg glute Bridges on the Wall with Single Leg Abduction
- 3 sets of 30 seconds each wall Planks with Side Plank Holds and Hip Dips

Day 16:

- Walking Squats on the Wall (3 sets of 10 repetitions per leg)
- Wall Side Plank with Leg Lifts and Twists (3 sets of 30 seconds)
- Preacher Curls on the Wall with Reverse Curls (3 sets of 12 repetitions)

- 3 sets of 12 repetitions of Wall Tricep Dips with Overhead Tricep Extensions and Diamond Push-Ups
- Wall Rows (3 sets of 12 repetitions)

Day 17:

- Holding a wall handstand with leg raises (3 sets of 30 seconds)
- V-Sit on the wall with single leg extensions (3 sets of 30 seconds each leg)
- Calf Raises on Toes and Wall Hamstring Curls using a Pilates Ball (3 sets x 12 repetitions each leg)
- Tuck Jumps with Wall Burpees (3 sets of 10 repetitions)

Week 6 & 7:

Continue with the exercises from Weeks 4 and 5, increasing the intensity progressively by:

- Increasing the amount of repetitions and sets.
- Reduce rest time between sets.
- Weights or resistance bands can be added.
- Experimenting with more complex forms of the workouts.

Week 8:

Day 28:

- Stretching and gentle aerobics for active recovery
- Celebrate your accomplishments and take stock of your development!

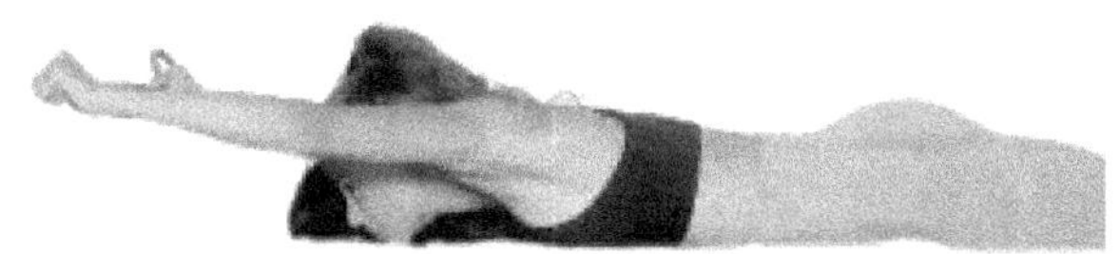

Additional Tips:

- Instead of focusing on speed, concentrate on perfect form.
- Throughout each workout, take deep breaths.
- Drink lots of water before, during, and after your workout to stay hydrated.
- To support your weight loss objectives, fuel your body with nutritious meals.
- Get enough sleep to allow your muscles to recuperate fully.
- Don't be scared to adapt workouts to your current fitness level.

- Have fun with the process!

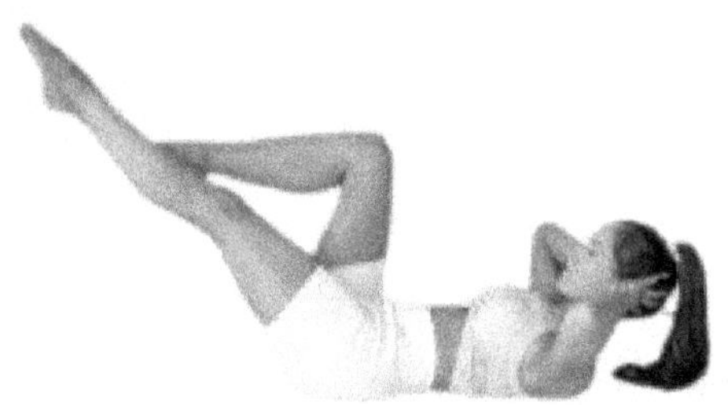

CHAPTER 5

Nutrition

Nutrition is important in weight loss since it influences:

Calorie intake: A calorie deficit is created by ingesting less calories than you burn, which is required for weight loss.

Hormones: The meals you consume have an effect on your hormones, which control appetite, satiety, and metabolism. The appropriate nutrients assist to balance these hormones, facilitating weight loss.

Energy levels: Eating healthy meals gives your body the energy it requires to power your exercises and everyday activities.

Muscle recovery: Proper nutrition provides your body with the building blocks it requires to repair and rebuild muscle tissue, allowing for speedier recovery and improving physical performance.

Overall health: A well-balanced diet rich in fruits, vegetables, whole grains, and lean protein promotes overall health by fortifying the immune system, increasing energy levels, and lowering the risk of chronic illnesses.

Healthy Weight Loss Eating Habits:

Prioritize fresh fruits and vegetables, whole grains, lean protein, and healthy fats above processed meals, sugary beverages, and refined carbs. These whole foods are naturally low in calories and high in vitamins, minerals, and fiber, which help you feel full and invigorated.

Control portion sizes: Be mindful of portion amounts to avoid overeating. Use measuring cups and spoons, eat mindfully, and pay attention to your body's hunger and fullness cues.

Include protein in every meal: Protein is necessary for muscle growth and maintenance, which helps to raise your metabolism and burn more calories. Include lean protein sources in each meal and snack, such as chicken, fish, beans, lentils, and tofu.

Choose good fats: good fats such as those found in avocados, nuts, seeds, and olive oil should not be avoided. These fats promote satiety, aid in hormone function, and improve general health.

Limit your intake of sugary drinks: Sugary drinks are high in empty calories and might lead to weight gain. Instead, drink water, unsweetened tea, or black coffee.

Plan your meals and snacks ahead of time: Planning your meals and snacks ahead of time allows you to make healthy choices when hunger strikes and avoids impulsive selections.

Check food labels: When selecting packaged goods, consider the serving size, calories, and ingredients. Choose selections that are fewer in calories, saturated fat, and added sugar.

Make healthy substitutions: Replace harmful foods with better options. For example, substitute whole-wheat bread for white bread, Greek yogurt for sour cream, and air-frying for deep-frying.

Cooking at home more regularly allows you to manage the contents and portion proportions of your meals. This enables you to prepare nutritious and tasty meals that support your weight loss objectives.

Don't starve yourself: Stay away from restricted diets and deprivation. To establish a healthy relationship with food and avoid binge eating, allow yourself occasional pleasures in moderation.

Drink enough of water: Drinking plenty of water throughout the day helps you feel full, increases metabolism, and promotes overall health. Aim for at least 8 glasses of water every day.

Meal Plan Ideas

Breakfast:

- (250 calories) Oatmeal with berries and nuts

- 1-piece whole-wheat bread with scrambled eggs (300 calories)
- (200 calories) Greek yogurt with fruit

Lunch:

- (400 calories) Salad with grilled chicken
- Tuna salad (300 calories) with whole-wheat crackers
- Dinner leftovers (400 calories)

Dinner:

(450 calories) Baked salmon with roasted veggies

Stir-fry chicken with brown rice (400 calories)

(350 calories) Lentil spaghetti with marinara sauce

Snacks:

- (200 calories) Apple with peanut butter
- (150 calories) Carrot sticks with hummus
- One small banana (100 calories).

Intermediate Level:

Breakfast:

- Protein powder, spinach, banana, and almond milk smoothie (300 calories)
- Pancakes made with whole wheat flour, fruit, and maple syrup (350 calories)
- (300 calories) Avocado toast with eggs

Lunch:

- (450 calories) Quinoa bowl with veggies and tofu
- (400 calories) Lentil soup with whole-wheat bread
- Sandwich of turkey on whole-wheat bread with avocado and lettuce (400 calories)

Dinner:

- Chili with turkey and cornbread (450 calories)
- (400 calories) Veggie burger on a whole-wheat baguette with sweet potato fries
- Scrambled tofu with veggies (350 calories)

Snacks:

- (200 calories) Cottage cheese with berries

- Eggs hard-boiled (150 calories)
- Avocado rice cakes (200 calories)

Advanced Level:

Breakfast:

- (250 calories) Greek yogurt with granola and berries
- Smoothie with spinach, banana, and almond milk (300 calories).
- 2 pieces whole-wheat bread with scrambled eggs (400 calories)

Lunch:

- Salad (500 calories) with grilled chicken or fish
- (500 calories) Quinoa bowl with veggies and nuts
- Dinner leftovers (500 calories)

Dinner:

- (550 calories) Baked salmon with roasted veggies
- Stir-fry chicken with brown rice and veggies (500 calories)
- (450 calories) Lentil spaghetti with marinara sauce and salad

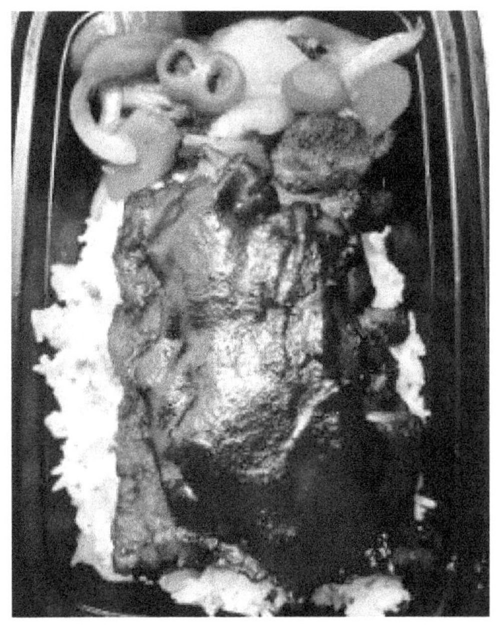

Snacks:

- (200 calories) Fruit with nuts and seeds
- (250 calories) Vegetables with hummus and whole-wheat crackers
- (250 calories) Cottage cheese with fruit and granola

NOTE

- These are simply exampling of meal plans; you may need to modify them to meet your own requirements and tastes.
- Consult a licensed dietitian or nutritionist for individualized advice and meal plans that are unique

to your weight reduction goals, health concerns, and
lifestyle.
*   Be adaptable and don't be scared to try new meals
    and dishes to find out what you like and what meets
    your budget and dietary limitations.
*   Most of all, enjoy your meals and concentrate on
    selecting good choices that feed your body and help
    you lose weight.

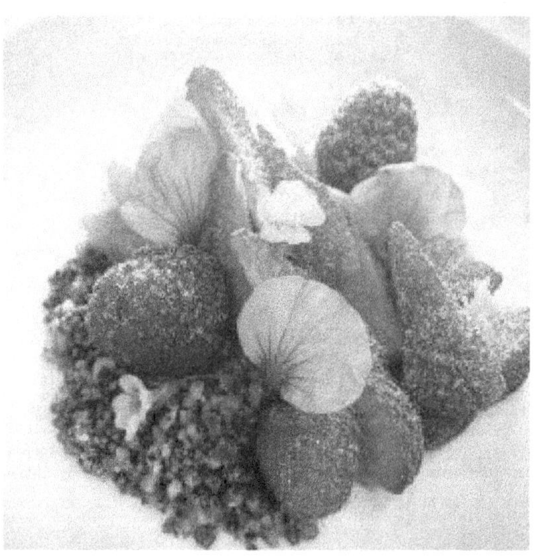

CHAPTTER 6

Adjust your calorie intake: To break through the plateau, reduce your calorie intake somewhat or increase your physical activity.

Incorporate new workouts or activities into your training program to push your body and muscles.

Strength training is important since it may boost your metabolism and help you burn more calories at rest.

Be patient: plateaus are typical and do not indicate failure. Maintain consistency and faith in the process.

Seek expert assistance: For specialized advice, speak with a licensed nutritionist or a professional personal trainer.

Avoiding Common Errors:

Setting unreasonable goals: Aiming for too much too soon might lead to disappointment and dissatisfaction. Set achievable targets and progressively raise the complexity as you go.

Avoid fad diets and excessively restricted eating behaviors. These diets are frequently unsustainable and can result in dietary shortages and poor food interactions.

Not keeping track of your progress: Keeping track of your food consumption and physical activity keeps you accountable and identifies areas for improvement.

Concentrating entirely on the scale's number: Weight loss is more than a metric. Consider your general health and energy levels, as well as how you feel and how your clothes fit.

Sleep deprivation: Getting adequate sleep is critical for weight reduction. To improve your metabolism and recuperation, aim for 7-8 hours of sleep every night.

Giving up after a setback: Everyone has difficulties along the way. Don't allow a single blunder stop your development. Get back on track and go on.

Making comparisons: Everyone's body and path are unique. Concentrate on your own success rather than comparing yourself to others.

CONCLUSION

Congratulations! You've arrived at the conclusion of your voyage via the realm of Wall Pilates for weight reduction. We've investigated the fundamentals, done the motions, and discovered the potential of this simple, effective workout. It's now time to flip the page and begin the next phase of your personal growth.

Note that Wall Pilates is not a fast remedy, but rather a long-term lifestyle change. It is all about developing a solid foundation of core strength, increasing flexibility, and learning to move your body with conscious control. These are the foundations of not only weight loss, but also total well-being.

Keep the following crucial points in mind as you proceed

Consistency reigns supreme (or queen!). Aim for at least 2-3 Wall Pilates sessions each week, or daily if possible. Keep in mind that little, consistent steps lead to large outcomes.

Pay attention to your body. Modify workouts as appropriate, and avoid pushing yourself too far. Enjoy the process and remember to enjoy every accomplishment, large or little.

Fuel your body correctly. A well-balanced meal is essential for optimizing your weight reduction potential and supporting your exercises. Eat healthful meals, remain hydrated, and pay attention to your hunger cues.

Accept the trip. Wall Pilates is about feeling stronger, more confident, and more in sync with your body, not just losing weight. Celebrate your non-scale triumphs, such as better posture, higher energy, and a fresh sense of control.

Remember that the wall is your companion, not your constraint. Wall Pilates may be your entryway to a stronger, leaner, and more powerful you with dedication and a little fun. So, take another step up to that wall, take a big breath, and let's keep pushing ahead together.

Keep it current! Explore new Wall Pilates variants and challenges as you advance. In this ever-changing discipline, there is always something new to learn and discover.

The final page is only the start of your narrative. Write your own success narrative in fitness, one Wall Pilates step at a time!

BONUS: WALL PILATE WORKOUT TRACKER

WEEKLY WALL PILATES WORKOUT PLAN

MON
TARGET ○ Full Body ○ Upper Body ○ Core ○ Lower Body ○ Active Rest

TUE
TARGET ○ Full Body ○ Upper Body ○ Core ○ Lower Body ○ Active Rest

WED
TARGET ○ Full Body ○ Upper Body ○ Core ○ Lower Body ○ Active Rest

THU
TARGET ○ Full Body ○ Upper Body ○ Core ○ Lower Body ○ Active Rest

FRI
TARGET ○ Full Body ○ Upper Body ○ Core ○ Lower Body ○ Active Rest

SAT
TARGET ○ Full Body ○ Upper Body ○ Core ○ Lower Body ○ Active Rest

SUN
TARGET ○ Full Body ○ Upper Body ○ Core ○ Lower Body ○ Active Rest

WEEKLY WALL PILATES WORKOUT PLAN

MON

TARGET ○ Full Body ○ Upper Body ○ Core ○ Lower Body ○ Active Rest

TUE

TARGET ○ Full Body ○ Upper Body ○ Core ○ Lower Body ○ Active Rest

WED

TARGET ○ Full Body ○ Upper Body ○ Core ○ Lower Body ○ Active Rest

THU

TARGET ○ Full Body ○ Upper Body ○ Core ○ Lower Body ○ Active Rest

FRI

TARGET ○ Full Body ○ Upper Body ○ Core ○ Lower Body ○ Active Rest

SAT

TARGET ○ Full Body ○ Upper Body ○ Core ○ Lower Body ○ Active Rest

SUN

TARGET ○ Full Body ○ Upper Body ○ Core ○ Lower Body ○ Active Rest

MON

TARGET ◯ Full Body ◯ Upper Body ◯ Core ◯ Lower Body ◯ Active Rest

TUE

TARGET ◯ Full Body ◯ Upper Body ◯ Core ◯ Lower Body ◯ Active Rest

WED

TARGET ◯ Full Body ◯ Upper Body ◯ Core ◯ Lower Body ◯ Active Rest

THU

TARGET ◯ Full Body ◯ Upper Body ◯ Core ◯ Lower Body ◯ Active Rest

FRI

TARGET ◯ Full Body ◯ Upper Body ◯ Core ◯ Lower Body ◯ Active Rest

SAT

TARGET ◯ Full Body ◯ Upper Body ◯ Core ◯ Lower Body ◯ Active Rest

SUN

TARGET ◯ Full Body ◯ Upper Body ◯ Core ◯ Lower Body ◯ Active Rest

WEEKLY WALL PILATES WORKOUT PLAN

MON
TARGET ◯ Full Body ◯ Upper Body ◯ Core ◯ Lower Body ◯ Active Rest

TUE
TARGET ◯ Full Body ◯ Upper Body ◯ Core ◯ Lower Body ◯ Active Rest

WED
TARGET ◯ Full Body ◯ Upper Body ◯ Core ◯ Lower Body ◯ Active Rest

THU
TARGET ◯ Full Body ◯ Upper Body ◯ Core ◯ Lower Body ◯ Active Rest

FRI
TARGET ◯ Full Body ◯ Upper Body ◯ Core ◯ Lower Body ◯ Active Rest

SAT
TARGET ◯ Full Body ◯ Upper Body ◯ Core ◯ Lower Body ◯ Active Rest

SUN
TARGET ◯ Full Body ◯ Upper Body ◯ Core ◯ Lower Body ◯ Active Rest

MON

TARGET ○ Full Body ○ Upper Body ○ Core ○ Lower Body ○ Active Rest

TUE

TARGET ○ Full Body ○ Upper Body ○ Core ○ Lower Body ○ Active Rest

WED

TARGET ○ Full Body ○ Upper Body ○ Core ○ Lower Body ○ Active Rest

THU

TARGET ○ Full Body ○ Upper Body ○ Core ○ Lower Body ○ Active Rest

FRI

TARGET ○ Full Body ○ Upper Body ○ Core ○ Lower Body ○ Active Rest

SAT

TARGET ○ Full Body ○ Upper Body ○ Core ○ Lower Body ○ Active Rest

SUN

TARGET ○ Full Body ○ Upper Body ○ Core ○ Lower Body ○ Active Rest

MON	**TARGET** ○ Full Body ○ Upper Body ○ Core ○ Lower Body ○ Active Rest
TUE	**TARGET** ○ Full Body ○ Upper Body ○ Core ○ Lower Body ○ Active Rest
WED	**TARGET** ○ Full Body ○ Upper Body ○ Core ○ Lower Body ○ Active Rest
THU	**TARGET** ○ Full Body ○ Upper Body ○ Core ○ Lower Body ○ Active Rest
FRI	**TARGET** ○ Full Body ○ Upper Body ○ Core ○ Lower Body ○ Active Rest
SAT	**TARGET** ○ Full Body ○ Upper Body ○ Core ○ Lower Body ○ Active Rest
SUN	**TARGET** ○ Full Body ○ Upper Body ○ Core ○ Lower Body ○ Active Rest

MON

TARGET ○ Full Body ○ Upper Body ○ Core ○ Lower Body ○ Active Rest

TUE

TARGET ○ Full Body ○ Upper Body ○ Core ○ Lower Body ○ Active Rest

WED

TARGET ○ Full Body ○ Upper Body ○ Core ○ Lower Body ○ Active Rest

THU

TARGET ○ Full Body ○ Upper Body ○ Core ○ Lower Body ○ Active Rest

FRI

TARGET ○ Full Body ○ Upper Body ○ Core ○ Lower Body ○ Active Rest

SAT

TARGET ○ Full Body ○ Upper Body ○ Core ○ Lower Body ○ Active Rest

SUN

TARGET ○ Full Body ○ Upper Body ○ Core ○ Lower Body ○ Active Rest

WEEKLY WALL PILATES WORKOUT PLAN

MON

TARGET ○ Full Body ○ Upper Body ○ Core ○ Lower Body ○ Active Rest

TUE

TARGET ○ Full Body ○ Upper Body ○ Core ○ Lower Body ○ Active Rest

WED

TARGET ○ Full Body ○ Upper Body ○ Core ○ Lower Body ○ Active Rest

THU

TARGET ○ Full Body ○ Upper Body ○ Core ○ Lower Body ○ Active Rest

FRI

TARGET ○ Full Body ○ Upper Body ○ Core ○ Lower Body ○ Active Rest

SAT

TARGET ○ Full Body ○ Upper Body ○ Core ○ Lower Body ○ Active Rest

SUN

TARGET ○ Full Body ○ Upper Body ○ Core ○ Lower Body ○ Active Rest

WEEKLY WALL PILATES WORKOUT PLAN

MON

TARGET ○ Full Body ○ Upper Body ○ Core ○ Lower Body ○ Active Rest

TUE

TARGET ○ Full Body ○ Upper Body ○ Core ○ Lower Body ○ Active Rest

WED

TARGET ○ Full Body ○ Upper Body ○ Core ○ Lower Body ○ Active Rest

THU

TARGET ○ Full Body ○ Upper Body ○ Core ○ Lower Body ○ Active Rest

FRI

TARGET ○ Full Body ○ Upper Body ○ Core ○ Lower Body ○ Active Rest

SAT

TARGET ○ Full Body ○ Upper Body ○ Core ○ Lower Body ○ Active Rest

SUN

TARGET ○ Full Body ○ Upper Body ○ Core ○ Lower Body ○ Active Rest

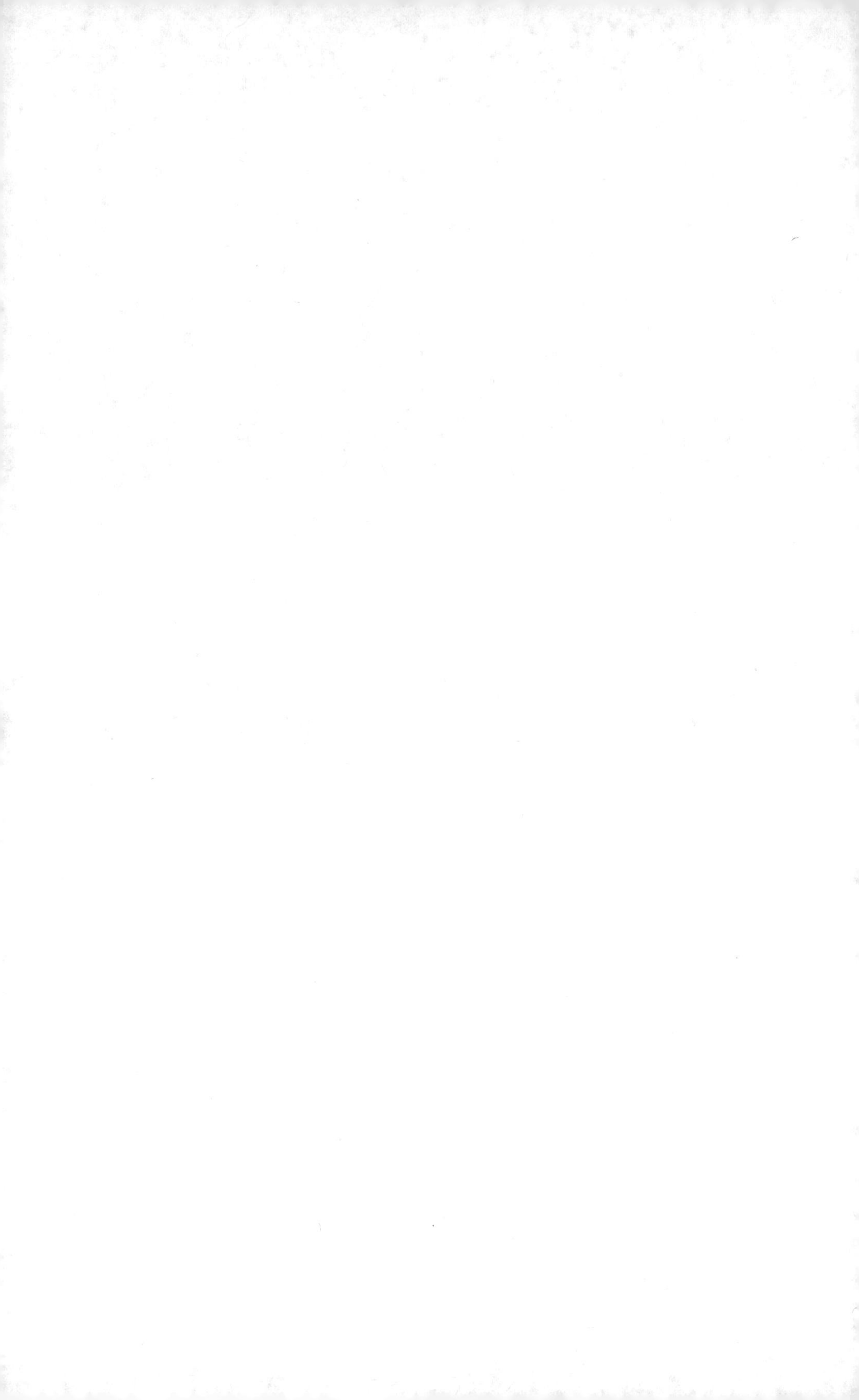